# THE NEW 2024 HCG DIET FOR BEGINNERS

The Super Easy Guide on How to Improve Insulin Resistance, Lose Weight Quickly, and Reset Body Your Body Metabolism Using 100+ Science-backed Diet Recipes

**Sarah Jordan LD, CCN**

# COPYRIGHT PAGE



The information and recipes in THE NEW 2024 HCG DIET FOR BEGINNERS: The Super Easy Guide on How to Improve Insulin Resistance, Lose Weight Quickly, and Reset Body Your Body Metabolism Using 100+ Science-backed Diet Recipes are not meant to replace professional medical or nutritional advice and are provided solely for educational reasons. The author and publisher disclaim all liability for any harm that may come from following the advice in this book. Before making any modifications to one's diet or beginning a program to lose weight, it is recommended that the reader seek the advice of a healthcare provider or nutritionist.

# Table of Contents

# Chapter 1: Understanding the HCG Diet

The Human Chorionic Gonadotropin (HCG) diet is a controversial and novel way to losing weight. Human chorionic gonadotropin (HCG) is a hormone that is generated by a pregnant woman's body. In the 1950s, a British endocrinologist named Dr. Albert Simeons developed the idea for the HCG diet.

This eating plan basically boils down to taking HCG in the form of injections or supplements and eating very few calories (between 500 and 800) per day. The basic premise is that HCG promotes the breakdown of stored fat for energy while protecting lean muscle mass, allowing for quick weight loss. As a result, the HCG diet has gained popularity, partly due to claims of great weight loss over a very short period.

However, it's important to note that the HCG diet has been met with some criticism and controversy from experts in the medical and nutritional fields. Skeptics say that the weight reduction observed during the HCG diet is mostly related to the rigorous calorie restriction rather than the HCG hormone itself.

Also, some people are worried that following such a low-calorie diet might lead to health problems including vitamin shortages and gallstones. Those who are looking for quick weight reduction solutions continue to be drawn to the HCG diet despite the controversy surrounding it.

Each phase of the HCG diet has its own set of nutritional requirements. These steps are meant to get the body ready, aid in weight reduction, and smoothly transition into a maintenance phase that will keep the weight off for good.

We'll discuss the research behind HCG, the diet's stages, some example meal plans, potential side effects, and other options for slimming down. We will also include first-hand stories from people who have successfully followed the HCG diet, providing a more complete picture of the program's advantages and disadvantages. While the HCG diet has shown promise for some, it should be used with caution and under the supervision of a healthcare expert who can assess your specific health and nutritional requirements.

## Background to the HCG

The HCG Diet's history reveals its beginnings and the conditions that prompted its creation. The notion of employing human chorionic gonadotropin (HCG) as a crucial component of a weight loss program was first proposed by British endocrinologist Dr. Albert Simeons in the 1950s.

Dr. Simeons first saw its benefits while treating pregnant mothers with malnutrition in India. Despite their low caloric consumption, he saw that these women gave birth to healthy infants, leading him to speculate that HCG had a role in rerouting nutrients from the mother's fat reserves to the developing infant.

The HCG Diet as we know it now may be traced back to Dr. Simeons's pioneering work in India. It was his hypothesis that an extremely low-calorie diet supplemented with HCG would cause the body to use its fat stores as a source of energy while protecting its lean muscle mass.

The HCG Diet program, based on this revolutionary theory, became popular in the 1950s and 1960s. The diet was made even more well-known when Dr. Simeons' book "Pounds and Inches: A New Approach to Obesity" was released.

The HCG Diet saw phases of popularity and decrease throughout the years, with different changes and adjustments to the original plan. Its rise in the early 21st century can be linked, in part, to increasing interest in alternative weight reduction procedures and a desire for speedy results.

The HCG Diet has a long history of popularity among individuals who want to lose weight rapidly, despite criticism and debate from medical and nutrition specialists.

Considerations of the HCG Diet's historical backdrop and the shifting viewpoints on its efficacy and safety are vital as we delve into its specifics. The history of the diet may tell us a lot about its evolution and its place among other weight reduction plans.

However, because to the significant calorie limits inherent in the HCG Diet, it is essential to approach the diet with an educated and cautious perspective, taking into account the potential hazards and the necessity for medical monitoring.

## What you Stand to Gain with the HCG Diet

The HCG Diet stands out from the crowd because of its singular goal and purported benefits, which have caught the interest of those in search of a quick and nontraditional means of losing weight. In order to evaluate the allure and possible success of this diet, it is crucial to grasp its key goals and anticipated rewards.

The HCG Diet is designed to promote quick and dramatic weight reduction. The diet is intended to help people lose weight rapidly, usually within a few weeks. Human chorionic gonadotropin (HCG), a hormone normally generated during pregnancy, and a severely limited daily caloric intake (between

500 and 800 calories) work together to accomplish this.

The hormone HCG has been shown to aid in the release of energy from fat stores while protecting valuable muscular tissue. The low-calorie diet aids in this procedure by producing a large calorie deficit, which in turn prompts the body to start breaking down stored fat for energy.

Proponents of the HCG Diet claim that among its advantages is significant weight reduction, often between 1 and 2 pounds each day. This is a major selling point for those trying to lose weight rapidly for reasons like getting in shape for a big event or getting their weight loss off to a good start.

Additionally, promoters of the HCG Diet say that it can lead to a reduction in body fat percentage, an improvement in body composition, and a boost in metabolism. Some people even say it can help them make healthier food choices in the long run by resetting their eating patterns.

The advantages of the HCG Diet, however, remain controversial among medical professionals and nutritionists. Some people think that the HCG hormone isn't responsible for the rapid weight loss seen on the diet, but rather that the rigorous calorie restriction involved.

In addition, they worry about vitamin shortages and the possibility of developing gallstones, both of which are linked to such a low-calorie diet. The advantages of the HCG Diet, notwithstanding these critiques, warrant thorough evaluation, ideally with the help of a healthcare practitioner.

In short, the HCG Diet's objective is to accomplish quick weight reduction by a combination of HCG treatment and a severely limited calorie diet. It is important to approach the diet with caution and informed decision making, taking into consideration the potential risks and seeking medical guidance when necessary, despite the fact that some people may experience the claimed benefits, such as fast and substantial weight loss, improved body composition, and metabolic changes.

# Chapter 2: The Science Backing HCG

Human Chorionic Gonadotropin (HCG) and its scientific basis in relation to the HCG Diet are intriguing and divisive topics. Insight into how this hormone is thought to affect the body's reaction to weight reduction may be gained by examining the underlying physiological mechanisms.

The placenta is responsible for the majority of HCG production throughout pregnancy, and this hormone is essential for fetal growth and development.

HCG diet advocates say the hormone makes it easier for the body to burn fat for fuel while protecting valuable muscular tissue. The hypothalamus, a part of the brain that regulates metabolism and other physical processes, is assumed to be the target of the hormone's effects.

The HCG Diet postulates that by resetting the hypothalamus, energy expenditures can be reduced and metabolic rate increased. This is considered to lessen sensations of hunger and exhaustion commonly associated with very low-calorie diets.

In addition, HCG is believed to provide a signal to the body to mobilize aberrant fat reserves, notably in the thighs, hips, and belly, to be used as fuel.

Proponents claim that, unlike with high calorie restriction diets, this approach leads to quick and considerable weight loss without the loss of muscle mass.

However, there is a lack of conclusive research to back up these claims, and the HCG Diet is still debated today. Some have argued that the HCG hormone is not responsible for the weight reduction that occurs on the HCG diet but rather that the extremely low calorie intake is to blame.

They say that there aren't enough high-quality clinical research linking HCG to weight loss to draw any firm conclusions. Nutritional deficits and gallstone development are only two of the health issues that have been identified as potential dangers of the diet.

The HCG Diet is supported by scientific evidence that centers on the hormone's alleged involvement in modulating the body's reaction to a very low-calorie diet.

The HCG diet is still controversial among medical professionals and nutritionists, despite claims by its proponents that it can aid in fat reduction while preserving muscle mass. It is crucial for those contemplating the HCG Diet to be aware of these concerns and approach it with carefully, ideally under the advice of a healthcare expert.

# Human Chorionic Gonadotropin (HCG)

The HCG Diet and its possible effects on the body can only be understood by first learning about Human Chorionic Gonadotropin (HCG). Understanding the physiological processes by which HCG performs its many important roles is essential for assessing the efficacy of the hormone in weight loss, especially during pregnancy.

Placental HCG (human chorionic gonadotropin) is a glycoprotein hormone that is essential to pregnancy and development. The corpus luteum is a transient endocrine structure in the ovaries whose main purpose is to sustain the developing fetus. A healthy uterine lining and early pregnancy depend on the hormone progesterone, which is produced with the help of this aid. Blood and urine HCG levels grow sharply in the first few weeks of pregnancy, providing the foundation for at-home pregnancy tests.

Proponents of the HCG Diet argue that HCG can affect the body's regulation of fat accumulation and energy consumption. They hypothesize that HCG influences the hypothalamus, which controls metabolism and food intake among other things in the body.

This idea proposes that HCG can improve the hypothalamus' capacity to utilize fat stores for energy, leading to weight reduction with minimal loss of muscle. The quick weight reduction achieved by the diet is thought to be due in part to this impact.

It should be noted, however, that the scientific proof for these claims is scant, and the HCG Diet continues to be debated. Weight reduction throughout the diet, critics say, is attributable more to the drastic calorie restriction than to the HCG itself.

Concerns have been raised about the possible health dangers involved with such intense calorie restriction, and there is a lack of robust clinical research proving a clear causal association between HCG and weight reduction.

Comprehending Human Chorionic Gonadotropin (HCG) entails realizing its function in sustaining pregnancy and appreciating its hypothesized affect on the hypothalamus within the framework of the HCG Diet.

Although HCG plays an important role in pregnancy and in regulating a number of other body processes, its ability to aid in weight loss is still up for discussion. Due to the lack of available scientific data and the possible hazards involved with the HCG Diet, anybody thinking about trying it is strongly advised to first visit a healthcare expert.

## HCG and its Effect on Your Body

Human Chorionic Gonadotropin (HCG) is a hormone generated during pregnancy, largely by cells in the placenta. It's gotten a lot of interest for its prospective medicinal and non-medical applications thanks to its pivotal involvement in a number of different physiological processes. The effects of HCG on the body are widespread, but they are more noticeable during pregnancy.

The transient endocrine structure known as the corpus luteum, which secretes progesterone, and the development of the placenta rely heavily on HCG's presence in early pregnancy.

Progesterone is essential because it helps keep the uterine lining healthy and aids in the growth of the fetus in its earliest stages. In the absence of HCG, the corpus luteum would atrophy, putting the pregnancy at danger.

During pregnancy, HCG is also crucial in regulating the body's metabolism. It's thought to aid in providing vital nutrients for the developing baby by encouraging the use of fat stores for energy, particularly in the first trimester. As a result, several weight reduction plans use HCG as a component since it can cause weight loss in pregnant women. However, the safety and efficacy of such programs are still a matter of dispute and inquiry.

HCG has received attention outside of pregnancy for its ability to increase testosterone levels in males. Because of this, it has found application in the therapy of hormonal disorders and in the promotion of conception.

HCG has also been used to improve athletic performance because of its ability to conceal the usage of anabolic steroids and other PEDs. There are now ethical and regulatory questions in the athletic world because of this.

Although HCG has several functions in the body, its primary and best-understood purpose is in sustaining the corpus luteum and fostering fetal development during pregnancy. The medical community is still debating and researching its various potential uses, including as in weight loss and hormone treatment.

Human chorionic gonadotropin (HCG) has important consequences for human health and well-being, making it crucial to understand its effects on the body for both clinical and non-medical uses.

## Controversies Surrounding the HCG Diet

The many uses of Human Chorionic Gonadotropin (HCG) and the claims made regarding its effects have made it the target of skepticism and debate.

Controversy surrounds the usage of HCG in weight loss methods like the HCG diet.

Concerns regarding HCG's safety and effectiveness have been raised by those who believe the hormone's effects on weight reduction are overstated and instead come from rigorous calorie restriction.

Many doctors are skeptical about the efficacy of HCG since the evidence for its usage outside of pregnancy is scant and conflicting. There is ongoing discussion on whether or not HCG is effective in certain settings.

The usage of HCG, which raises testosterone levels and hence improves athletic performance, raises ethical questions in the sports industry. Such techniques are considered immoral and unlawful, potentially providing athletes an undue edge and breaking anti-doping laws.

The debate is on the off-label usage of HCG, or the use of a drug outside of its approved medical context. Critics warn against untested uses of HCG, claiming that these applications may lack enough control and regulation and highlighting the need of evidence-based medicine.

Safety issues also exist, since some persons may have unpleasant effects including headaches, lethargy, and edema when utilizing HCG for various causes. Another area of worry is the safety of using HCG for extended periods of time, especially in weight loss regimens.

Because of differences in HCG regulation and monitoring from one nation to the next, the quality and safety of HCG products on the market might vary widely. Consumers may find it difficult to make well-informed decisions concerning HCG-based therapy due to this lack of uniformity. Although HCG has been shown to have beneficial medicinal effects in helping mothers through pregnancy, its off-label usage have been met with skepticism and discussion.

Potential patients using HCG-based therapies should discuss their options with their doctors, learn about the hazards involved, and weigh the benefits against them before making any decisions.

The HCG diet is a multi-stage regimen designed to help people shed excess pounds. Human chorionic gonadotropin (HCG) is a hormone that works in tandem with these stages to aid in weight loss. The HCG diet typically consists of the following stages:

## Phase 1: Loading

The average duration is two days. At this point, it's recommended that people eat a lot of high-calorie, high-fat meals in order to bulk up. This phase helps prepare the body for the low-calorie period that follows.

## Phase 2: the Low-Calorie Stage

The average duration is between 21 and 40 days. Phase 2 of the HCG diet is where the magic happens. Participants use HCG drops or injectables while adhering to a very low-calorie diet of 500 to 800 calories per day.

It is thought that the HCG hormone aids the body in breaking down fat reserves for fuel without causing any significant muscle loss. This is supposed to help you shed pounds quickly.

Dietary restrictions often involve eating fewer calories and fewer items high in fat and sugar. The diet frequently contains lean meats, veggies, and limited fruit.

## Phase 3: Maintenance

This phase often lasts for three weeks. After the low-calorie period is over, individuals maintain their low-calorie diet for a few more days without the hormone HCG. The weight reduction is steadier this way.

Normal foods are reintroduced gradually, although carbs and sweets are restricted at first. During this stage, the emphasis is on staying within a healthy weight range. Better nutritional habits might also be formed throughout this period.

## Phase 4: Stabilization

The timeframe is normally three weeks. In this phase, individuals continue to concentrate on regulating their weight. It's crucial to keep the new weight stable and not let it go back to the old one. Participants return a wider variety of foods to their diet over time, however they should continue to exercise restraint when it comes to high-calorie or processed options.

## Phase 5: The Transition

The transition phase is essentially a lifelong commitment to healthy eating and preserving the weight loss accomplished during the HCG diet. Making healthy food choices and maintaining an active lifestyle might help you keep the weight off.

The HCG diet's efficacy and safety are hotly debated amongst medical professionals, so it's vital to keep that in mind.

Extreme calorie restriction and the use of HCG for weight reduction have been met with skepticism by many medical professionals and organizations, including the FDA in the United States. Potential hazards and advantages of this diet should be discussed with a doctor before beginning.

## Foods to Consider on the HCG Diet

The HCG diet is an extremely stringent eating plan that involves eating just certain foods and cutting out many others.

The diet is often separated into phases, and the permissible items may vary significantly dependent on the exact protocol being followed. The HCG diet normally permits the following foods:

**Lean Proteins:**

- Skinless chicken breast
- Lean cuts of beef (e.g., sirloin, tenderloin)
- White fish (e.g., tilapia, cod, haddock)
- Shrimp
- Crab
- Turkey
- Game meats (e.g., bison, venison)

**Vegetables**

- Spinach

- Lettuce (green leaf, romaine)

- Cabbage

- Tomatoes (in limited quantities)

- Asparagus

- Cucumbers

- Celery

- Broccoli

- Cauliflower

- Green beans

**Fruits (in very limited quantities)**

- Apples

- Strawberries

- Oranges (usually only in small amounts)

**Beverages**

- Water (encouraged for hydration)

- Herbal teas (caffeine-free)

- Black coffee (in moderation, without added sugar or high-fat cream)

**Seasonings and Spices (used sparingly)**

- Salt

- Pepper

- Garlic

- Basil

- Thyme

- Parsley

- Mustard

- Apple cider vinegar (as a salad dressing)

During the low-calorie phase of the HCG diet, calorie intake is tightly restricted to roughly 500 to 800 calories per day, and portion sizes are rigorously managed. The goal is to promote fat loss while keeping your muscle mass intact, thus a diet low in both carbs and fat is emphasized.

The HCG diet prohibits the eating of high-calorie and high-fat foods, such as oils, butter, dairy, and sweet goods. Breads, pastas, and cereals are often not allowed either.

The HCG diet is a highly contentious weight reduction treatment, and its safety and efficacy are issues of discussion; thus, it is important to speak with a healthcare expert before beginning the diet. Extreme calorie restriction isn't healthy for everyone and comes with its own set of hazards.

# Foods to Avoid on the HCG Diet

To lose weight on the HCG diet, dieters must strictly adhere to a list of prohibited items. The emphasis is on lowering calorie consumption and banning particular types of foods that are considered to interfere with the diet's efficacy. On the HCG diet, you should stay away from meals like these:

## High-Fat Meats

- Fatty cuts of beef (e.g., ribeye, T-bone)
- Pork
- Lamb
- Sausages
- Bacon

## Dairy Products

- Milk

- Cheese

- Yogurt

- Butter

## Oils and Fats

- Cooking oils (e.g., olive oil, coconut oil)

- Salad dressings

- Margarine

- Mayonnaise

## High-Carb Foods

- Bread

- Pasta

- Rice

- Cereals

- Grains

- Legumes (e.g., beans, lentils)

## Sugary and Processed Foods

- Sugary snacks and desserts
- Candy
- Chips
- Fast food
- Processed foods with added sugars and fats

## Nuts and Seeds

- Almonds
- Peanuts
- Sunflower seeds
- Cashews

## Beverages

- Alcohol
- Fruit juices
- Soft drinks and soda

- High-calorie coffee drinks

## High-Carb Vegetables

- Potatoes
- Corn
- Peas
- Carrots
- Beets

## High-Fat Condiments

- Mayonnaise
- Salad dressings with oil
- Sour cream

## High-Sugar Fruits

- Bananas
- Grapes

- Mangoes

- Cherries

The HCG diet emphasizes lean proteins and low-carb, low-fat, and low-sugar alternatives while limiting calorie intake and the sorts of foods allowed. High-calorie and high-fat foods should be avoided as much as possible in order to produce a big calorie deficit and encourage weight reduction.

It's worth noting that the HCG diet is a contentious method of losing weight, with many people questioning both its safety and efficacy. Before commencing on this diet, it's essential to speak with a healthcare practitioner to understand the potential dangers and advantages and to confirm that it is an appropriate choice for specific weight reduction goals and health concerns.

# A 2 Day Sample Meal on the HCG Diet

The HCG diet calls for strict adherence to a regimen of three daily modest, low-calorie meals. These dishes are planned to provide all the nutrients your body needs at very low calorie counts. Those on the HCG diet are required to adhere to a strict eating plan. An example HCG diet menu is as follows:

**Day 1**

**Breakfast:**

- Grilled chicken breast (3.5 ounces)
- Steamed asparagus (1 cup)
- Herbal tea or black coffee (no sugar or cream)

## Lunch:

- Whitefish (3.5 ounces)
- Mixed greens (e.g., lettuce, spinach) with apple cider vinegar as dressing
- A small apple

## Dinner:

- Lean beef (3.5 ounces)
- Steamed broccoli (1 cup)
- Herbal tea or black coffee

## Day 2

## Breakfast:

- Turkey breast (3.5 ounces)

- Sliced cucumber (1 cup)

- Herbal tea or black coffee (no sugar or cream)

## Lunch

- Shrimp (3.5 ounces)

- Mixed greens with apple cider vinegar dressing

- A small orange

## Dinner

- Chicken breast (3.5 ounces)

- Sliced zucchini (1 cup)

- Herbal tea or black coffee

## BREAKFAST RECIPES

### Spinach and Mushroom Omelette

*Nutritional Information (Approximate):*

Calories: 75

Protein: 12g

Carbohydrates: 4g

Fat: 0g

**Ingredients**

3 egg whites

1 cup fresh spinach

1/4 cup sliced mushrooms

Salt and pepper to taste

**Instructions**

Whisk the egg whites in a bowl.

Heat a non-stick skillet over medium heat.

Add spinach and mushrooms to the skillet and cook until they start to wilt.

Pour the whisked egg whites over the vegetables.

Cook until the omelette is set and the edges are lightly browned.

Season with salt and pepper and fold the omelette in half.

## Greek Yogurt with Berries

*Nutritional Information (Approximate):*

Calories: 120

Protein: 10g

Carbohydrates: 15g

Fat: 1g

**Ingredients**

1/2 cup plain Greek yogurt

1/2 cup mixed berries (e.g., strawberries, blueberries)

**Instructions**

Place Greek yogurt in a bowl.

Top with mixed berries.

Optional: Drizzle with a few drops of stevia or a sprinkle of cinnamon for added flavor.

## Cottage Cheese and Pineapple

*Nutritional Information (Approximate):*

Calories: 125

Protein: 14g

Carbohydrates: 18g

Fat: 1g

## Ingredients

1/2 cup low-fat cottage cheese

1/2 cup fresh pineapple chunks

## Instructions

Combine cottage cheese and pineapple in a bowl.

Vegetable Scramble

*Nutritional Information (Approximate):*

Calories: 80

Protein: 14g

Carbohydrates: 5g

Fat: 0g

**Ingredients**

3 egg whites

1/4 cup diced bell peppers (assorted colors)

1/4 cup diced onions

1/4 cup diced tomatoes

Salt and pepper to taste

**Instructions**

Whisk the egg whites in a bowl.

In a non-stick skillet, sauté the diced vegetables until tender.

Pour the egg whites over the vegetables.

Cook, stirring gently, until the eggs are fully set. Season with salt and pepper.

## Apple and Cinnamon Oatmeal

*Nutritional Information (Approximate):*
Calories: 110

Protein: 3g

Carbohydrates: 24g

Fat: 1g

**Ingredients**

1/4 cup rolled oats

1/2 small apple, diced

A dash of cinnamon

Stevia (optional, for added sweetness)

**Instructions**

Cook the oats according to package instructions, using water.

Stir in diced apples, cinnamon, and stevia, if desired.

## Smoked Salmon Lettuce Wraps

### Nutritional Information (Approximate):

Calories: 100

Protein: 14g

Carbohydrates: 2g

Fat: 4g

## Ingredients

2 oz smoked salmon

Lettuce leaves (e.g., Romaine or Butterhead)

1/4 cup diced cucumbers

1/4 cup diced tomatoes

Dill (for garnish)

Lemon wedges (optional)

**Instructions**

Lay the smoked salmon slices on lettuce leaves.

Top with diced cucumbers and tomatoes.

Garnish with dill and a squeeze of lemon, if desired.

## Spinach and Tomato Breakfast Wrap

*Nutritional Information (Approximate):*

Calories: 90

Protein: 14g

Carbohydrates: 7g

Fat: 0g

## Ingredients

3 egg whites

1 cup fresh spinach

1/2 cup diced tomatoes

Salt and pepper to taste

## Instructions

Whisk the egg whites in a bowl.

Heat a non-stick skillet over medium heat.

Add spinach and tomatoes to the skillet and cook
until wilted.

Pour the whisked egg whites over the vegetables.

Cook until the eggs are set. Season with salt and
pepper.

Roll the egg and vegetable mixture in a lettuce leaf
or a large cabbage leaf to create a wrap.

## Berry Smoothie

*Nutritional Information (Approximate):*

Calories: 100

Protein: 10g

Carbohydrates: 18g

Fat: 1g

## Ingredients

1/2 cup mixed berries (e.g., strawberries, blueberries)

1/2 cup unsweetened almond milk

1/2 cup ice

Stevia (optional, for added sweetness)

**Instructions**

Combine mixed berries, almond milk, ice, and stevia in a blender.

Blend until smooth.

## Avocado and Tomato Salad

*Nutritional Information (Approximate):*

Calories: 140

Protein: 2g

Carbohydrates: 10g

Fat: 10g

## Ingredients

1/2 avocado, diced

1/2 cup diced tomatoes

1/4 cup diced onions

Cilantro (for garnish)

Salt and pepper to taste

## Instructions

Combine diced avocado, tomatoes, and onions in a bowl.

Season with salt and pepper.

Garnish with fresh cilantro.

## Asparagus and Tomato Breakfast Skillet

*Nutritional Information (Approximate):*

Calories: 85

Protein: 4g

Carbohydrates: 12g

Fat: 3g

**Ingredients**

1/2 cup asparagus spears

1/2 cup diced tomatoes

1/4 cup diced onions

3 egg whites

Salt and pepper to taste

**Instructions**

Heat a non-stick skillet over medium heat.

Add asparagus, tomatoes, and onions to the skillet and sauté until tender.

Whisk the egg whites in a bowl and pour them over the vegetables.

Cook until the eggs are set. Season with salt and pepper.

# Veggie and Turkey Sausage Scramble

*Nutritional Information (Approximate):*

Calories: 120

Protein: 15g

Carbohydrates: 4g

Fat: 5g

## Ingredients

3 egg whites

2 oz cooked turkey sausage (crumbled)

1/4 cup diced bell peppers (assorted colors)

1/4 cup diced onions

Salt and pepper to taste

**Instructions**

Whisk the egg whites in a bowl.

In a non-stick skillet, cook the crumbled turkey sausage until heated through.

Add bell peppers and onions and sauté until tender.

Pour the whisked egg whites over the sausage and vegetables.

Cook, stirring gently, until the eggs are fully set. Season with salt and pepper.

# Berries and Cottage Cheese Bowl

*Nutritional Information (Approximate):*

Calories: 120

Protein: 14g

Carbohydrates: 12g

Fat: 2g

## Ingredients

1/2 cup low-fat cottage cheese

1/2 cup mixed berries (e.g., blueberries, raspberries)

Stevia (optional, for added sweetness)

## Instructions

Place low-fat cottage cheese in a bowl.

Top with mixed berries.

Optional: Drizzle with a few drops of stevia for added sweetness.

## Egg and Spinach Breakfast Wrap

*Nutritional Information (Approximate):*

Calories: 90

Protein: 12g

Carbohydrates: 6g

Fat: 3g

**Ingredients**

3 egg whites

1 cup fresh spinach

Salt and pepper to taste

A lettuce leaf or cabbage leaf for wrapping

**Instructions**

Whisk the egg whites in a bowl.

Heat a non-stick skillet over medium heat.

Add spinach to the skillet and cook until wilted.

Pour the whisked egg whites over the spinach.

Cook until the eggs are set. Season with salt and pepper.

Roll the egg and spinach mixture in a lettuce or cabbage leaf to create a wrap.

## Chia Seed Pudding

*Nutritional Information (Approximate):*

Calories: 100

Protein: 4g

Carbohydrates: 10g

Fat: 5g

# Ingredients

2 tbsp chia seeds

1/2 cup unsweetened almond milk

Stevia (optional, for added sweetness)

Berries (optional, for topping)

# Instructions

Combine chia seeds and almond milk in a bowl.

Stir well and refrigerate for several hours or overnight to allow the pudding to thicken.

Add stevia for sweetness and top with berries if desired.

## Smoked Turkey and Asparagus Frittata

*Nutritional Information (Approximate):*

Calories: 130

Protein: 15g

Carbohydrates: 4g

Fat: 6g

## Ingredients

3 egg whites

2 oz smoked turkey, chopped

1/2 cup asparagus spears, chopped

Salt and pepper to taste

**Instructions**

Whisk the egg whites in a bowl.

Preheat the broiler in your oven.

In an oven-safe skillet, sauté the chopped smoked turkey and asparagus until tender.

Pour the whisked egg whites over the turkey and asparagus.

Cook on the stovetop until the edges start to set.

Place the skillet under the broiler for a few minutes to finish cooking the frittata.

Season with salt and pepper.

# Zucchini and Tomato Omelette

*Nutritional Information (Approximate):*

Calories: 80

Protein: 10g

Carbohydrates: 4g

Fat: 3g

## Ingredients

3 egg whites

1/4 cup diced zucchini

1/4 cup diced tomatoes

Salt and pepper to taste

**Instructions**

Whisk the egg whites in a bowl.

Heat a non-stick skillet over medium heat.

Add zucchini and tomatoes to the skillet and cook until the zucchini is tender.

Pour the whisked egg whites over the vegetables.

Cook until the omelette is set. Season with salt and pepper.

**Strawberry Protein Smoothie**

*Nutritional Information (Approximate):*

Calories: 120

Protein: 15g

Carbohydrates: 15g

Fat: 1g

**Ingredients**

1/2 cup frozen strawberries

1/2 cup unsweetened almond milk

1/2 scoop vanilla protein powder

Stevia (optional, for added sweetness)

**Instructions**

Combine frozen strawberries, almond milk, and protein powder in a blender.

Blend until smooth.

Add stevia for sweetness if desired.

## Broccoli and Tomato Breakfast Skillet

*Nutritional Information (Approximate)*

Calories: 90

Protein: 8g

Carbohydrates: 10g

Fat: 2g

**Ingredients**

1/2 cup broccoli florets

1/2 cup diced tomatoes

3 egg whites

Salt and pepper to taste

**Instructions**

Heat a non-stick skillet over medium heat.

Add broccoli and tomatoes to the skillet and sauté until tender.

Whisk the egg whites in a bowl and pour them over the vegetables.

Cook until the eggs are set. Season with salt and pepper.

## Tuna Salad Lettuce Wraps

*Nutritional Information (Approximate):*

Calories: 130

Protein: 16g

Carbohydrates: 2g

Fat: 6g

**Ingredients**

3 oz canned tuna in water, drained

Lettuce leaves (e.g., Romaine or Butterhead)

1/4 cup diced celery

1/4 cup diced onions

Lemon juice (for flavor)

Salt and pepper to taste

**Instructions**

In a bowl, combine drained tuna, diced celery, diced onions, and a squeeze of lemon juice.

Season with salt and pepper.

Spoon the tuna salad onto lettuce leaves to create wraps.

# Cucumber and Dill Cottage Cheese

*Nutritional Information (Approximate):*

Calories: 110

Protein: 14g

Carbohydrates: 8g

Fat: 2g

**Ingredients**

1/2 cup low-fat cottage cheese

1/2 cup sliced cucumber

Fresh dill (for garnish)

Salt and pepper to taste

## Instructions

Combine low-fat cottage cheese and sliced cucumber in a bowl.

Season with salt and pepper.

Garnish with fresh dill.

# LUNCH RECIPES

## Grilled Chicken Salad

*Nutritional Information (Approximate):*

Calories: 150

Protein: 25g

Carbohydrates: 4g

Fat: 4g

**Ingredients**

3 oz grilled chicken breast

2 cups mixed greens (e.g., spinach, arugula)

1/4 cup cherry tomatoes

1/4 cup cucumber slices

Balsamic vinegar (as dressing)

**Instructions**

Grill the chicken breast until fully cooked.

Slice the grilled chicken into thin strips.

Combine mixed greens, cherry tomatoes, and cucumber in a bowl.

Top with grilled chicken strips and drizzle with balsamic vinegar.

# Shrimp and Asparagus Stir-Fry

*Nutritional Information (Approximate):*

Calories: 160

Protein: 25g

Carbohydrates: 5g

Fat: 4g

## Ingredients

3 oz cooked shrimp

1/2 cup asparagus spears, cut into bite-sized pieces

1/4 cup sliced bell peppers (assorted colors)

1/4 cup diced onions

1 clove garlic, minced

Low-sodium soy sauce (for flavor)

**Instructions**

Heat a non-stick skillet over medium heat.

Add asparagus, bell peppers, onions, and garlic to the skillet and sauté until tender.

Add the cooked shrimp and a dash of low-sodium soy sauce.

Stir-fry for a few minutes until heated through.

# Turkey and Cucumber Wrap

*Nutritional Information (Approximate):*

Calories: 120

Protein: 20g

Carbohydrates: 4g

Fat: 2g

## Ingredients

3 oz lean ground turkey, cooked and seasoned

1 large cucumber, peeled into thin strips

1/4 cup diced tomatoes

Lettuce leaves (e.g., Romaine or Butterhead)

## Instructions

Season and cook the lean ground turkey until fully cooked.

Place cucumber strips on lettuce leaves.

Top with cooked ground turkey and diced tomatoes.

Roll the lettuce leaves to create wraps.


## Grilled White Fish with Steamed Broccoli

*Nutritional Information (Approximate):*

Calories: 140

Protein: 25g

Carbohydrates: 4g

Fat: 2g

**Ingredients**

3 oz grilled white fish (e.g., tilapia or cod)

1 cup steamed broccoli florets

Lemon juice (for flavor)

Salt and pepper to taste

**Instructions**

Grill the white fish until fully cooked.

Season with lemon juice, salt, and pepper.

Serve with steamed broccoli on the side.

## Cabbage and Ground Beef Stir-Fry

*Nutritional Information (Approximate):*

Calories: 160

Protein: 20g

Carbohydrates: 10g

Fat: 5g

## Ingredients

3 oz lean ground beef

1 cup shredded cabbage

1/4 cup diced onions

1/4 cup diced bell peppers (assorted colors)

Low-sodium soy sauce (for flavor)

**Instructions**

In a non-stick skillet, cook the lean ground beef until fully cooked.

Add cabbage, onions, and bell peppers to the skillet and sauté until tender.

Add a dash of low-sodium soy sauce for flavor.

## Spinach and Strawberry Salad

*Nutritional Information (Approximate):*

Calories: 140

Protein: 6g

Carbohydrates: 12g

Fat: 7g

**Ingredients**

2 cups fresh spinach

1/2 cup sliced strawberries

2 tbsp slivered almonds

Balsamic vinegar (as dressing)

**Instructions**

Combine fresh spinach, sliced strawberries, and slivered almonds in a bowl.

Drizzle with balsamic vinegar for dressing.

## Baked Chicken and Asparagus

*Nutritional Information (Approximate):*

Calories: 150

Protein: 25g

Carbohydrates: 4g

Fat: 3g

## Ingredients

3 oz boneless, skinless chicken breast

1/2 cup asparagus spears

Lemon juice (for flavor)

Salt and pepper to taste

## Instructions

Preheat the oven to 375°F (190°C).

Place chicken breast and asparagus on a baking sheet.

Season with lemon juice, salt, and pepper.

Bake until the chicken is fully cooked and the asparagus is tender.

# Ground Turkey and Zucchini Skillet

*Nutritional Information (Approximate):*

Calories: 140

Protein: 20g

Carbohydrates: 6g

Fat: 5g

## Ingredients

3 oz lean ground turkey

1/2 cup diced zucchini

1/4 cup diced tomatoes

1/4 cup diced onions

1 clove garlic, minced

Salt and pepper to taste

**Instructions**

In a non-stick skillet, cook the lean ground turkey until fully cooked.

Add zucchini, tomatoes, onions, and garlic to the skillet and sauté until tender.

Season with salt and pepper.

**Tofu and Spinach Stir-Fry**

*Nutritional Information (Approximate):*

Calories: 150

Protein: 15g

Carbohydrates: 10g

Fat: 6g

**Ingredients**

4 oz extra-firm tofu, cubed

1 cup fresh spinach

1/4 cup sliced mushrooms

1/4 cup diced bell peppers (assorted colors)

Low-sodium soy sauce (for flavor)

**Instructions**

In a non-stick skillet, cook the tofu until heated through.

Add spinach, mushrooms, and bell peppers to the skillet and sauté until tender.

Add a dash of low-sodium soy sauce for flavor.

## Spaghetti Squash with Marinara Sauce

*Nutritional Information (Approximate):*

Calories: 120

Protein: 2g

Carbohydrates: 14g

Fat: 6g

**Ingredients**

1 cup cooked spaghetti squash

1/2 cup sugar-free marinara sauce

Fresh basil (for garnish)

Salt and pepper to taste

**Instructions**

Cook the spaghetti squash until tender and scrape the strands with a fork.

Heat sugar-free marinara sauce and pour it over the spaghetti squash.

Season with salt and pepper.

Garnish with fresh basil.

## Lemon Garlic Shrimp with Asparagus

*Nutritional Information (Approximate):*

Calories: 150

Protein: 25g

Carbohydrates: 5g

Fat: 4g

## Ingredients

3 oz cooked shrimp

1/2 cup asparagus spears

1 clove garlic, minced

Juice of half a lemon

Salt and pepper to taste

## Instructions

In a non-stick skillet, sauté the cooked shrimp, asparagus, and minced garlic until heated through.

Squeeze lemon juice over the mixture and season with salt and pepper.

# Cucumber and Tuna Salad

## *Nutritional Information (Approximate):*

Calories: 130

Protein: 20g

Carbohydrates: 6g

Fat: 2g

## Ingredients

3 oz canned tuna in water, drained

1 large cucumber, diced

1/4 cup diced tomatoes

1/4 cup diced onions

Lemon juice (for flavor)

Salt and pepper to taste

**Instructions**

In a bowl, combine drained tuna, diced cucumber, diced tomatoes, and diced onions.

Season with lemon juice, salt, and pepper.

## Turkey and Spinach Salad

*Nutritional Information (Approximate):*

Calories: 150

Protein: 20g

Carbohydrates: 5g

Fat: 5g

**Ingredients**

3 oz cooked and sliced turkey breast

2 cups fresh spinach

1/4 cup sliced strawberries

2 tbsp slivered almonds

Balsamic vinegar (as dressing)

**Instructions**

Place sliced turkey breast on a bed of fresh spinach.

Top with sliced strawberries and slivered almonds.

Drizzle with balsamic vinegar for dressing.

## Beef and Broccoli Stir-Fry

*Nutritional Information (Approximate):*

Calories: 160

Protein: 20g

Carbohydrates: 8g

Fat: 6g

**Ingredients**

3 oz lean beef strips

1/2 cup broccoli florets

1/4 cup diced onions

1/4 cup sliced mushrooms

Low-sodium soy sauce (for flavor)

**Instructions**

In a non-stick skillet, cook the lean beef strips until fully cooked.

Add broccoli, onions, and mushrooms to the skillet and sauté until tender.

Add a dash of low-sodium soy sauce for flavor.

# Tofu and Vegetable Stir-Fry

*Nutritional Information (Approximate):*

Calories: 140

Protein: 15g

Carbohydrates: 10g

Fat: 6g

## Ingredients

4 oz extra-firm tofu, cubed

1/2 cup sliced bell peppers (assorted colors)

1/2 cup sliced zucchini

1/4 cup diced onions

Low-sodium soy sauce (for flavor)

**Instructions**

In a non-stick skillet, cook the tofu until heated through.

Add bell peppers, zucchini, onions, and a dash of low-sodium soy sauce.

Sauté until vegetables are tender.

## Mixed Greens with Grilled Chicken

*Nutritional Information (Approximate):*

Calories: 150

Protein: 25g

Carbohydrates: 4g

Fat: 4g

**Ingredients**

3 oz grilled chicken breast, sliced

2 cups mixed greens (e.g., arugula, Romaine)

1/4 cup cherry tomatoes

1/4 cup sliced cucumbers

Lemon vinaigrette (as dressing)

**Instructions**

Place sliced grilled chicken on a bed of mixed greens.

Top with cherry tomatoes and sliced cucumbers.

Drizzle with lemon vinaigrette for dressing.

## Turkey and Zucchini Noodles

*Nutritional Information (Approximate):*

Calories: 140

Protein: 20g

Carbohydrates: 6g

Fat: 5g

## Ingredients

3 oz lean ground turkey, cooked and seasoned

1 zucchini, spiralized into noodles

1/4 cup diced tomatoes

1/4 cup diced onions

Salt and pepper to taste

## Instructions

Season and cook the lean ground turkey until fully cooked.

In a skillet, sauté zucchini noodles, diced tomatoes, and diced onions until heated through.

Top with cooked ground turkey and season with salt and pepper.

## Baked White Fish with Steamed Asparagus

*Nutritional Information (Approximate):*

Calories: 140

Protein: 25g

Carbohydrates: 4g

Fat: 3g

**Ingredients**

3 oz white fish (e.g., tilapia or cod)

1 cup steamed asparagus spears

Lemon juice (for flavor)

Salt and pepper to taste

**Instructions**

Bake the white fish until fully cooked.

Season with lemon juice, salt, and pepper.

Serve with steamed asparagus on the side.

## Cabbage and Shrimp Stir-Fry

*Nutritional Information (Approximate):*

Calories: 160

Protein: 25g

Carbohydrates: 10g

Fat: 4g

**Ingredients**

3 oz cooked shrimp

1 cup shredded cabbage

1/4 cup diced onions

1/4 cup sliced bell peppers (assorted colors)

Low-sodium soy sauce (for flavor)

**Instructions**

In a non-stick skillet, sauté the cooked shrimp, shredded cabbage, diced onions, and sliced bell peppers until heated through.

Add a dash of low-sodium soy sauce for flavor.

## Avocado and Tomato Salad

*Nutritional Information (Approximate):*

Calories: 140

Protein: 2g

Carbohydrates: 10g

Fat: 10g

## Ingredients

1/2 avocado, diced

1/2 cup diced tomatoes

1/4 cup diced onions

Fresh cilantro (for garnish)

Salt and pepper to taste

## Instructions

Combine diced avocado, diced tomatoes, and diced onions in a bowl.

Season with salt and pepper.

Garnish with fresh cilantro.

# DINNER RECIPES

## Lemon Garlic Grilled Chicken

*Nutritional Information (Approximate):*

Calories: 150

Protein: 25g

Carbohydrates: 2g

Fat: 4g

**Ingredients**

4 oz grilled chicken breast

1 clove garlic, minced

Juice of half a lemon

Salt and pepper to taste

**Instructions**

Grill the chicken breast until fully cooked.

Season with minced garlic, lemon juice, salt, and pepper.

## Baked Tilapia with Roasted Asparagus

*Nutritional Information (Approximate):*

Calories: 140

Protein: 25g

Carbohydrates: 4g

Fat: 3g

**Ingredients**

4 oz tilapia fillet

1 cup roasted asparagus spears

Lemon juice (for flavor)

Salt and pepper to taste

**Instructions**

Preheat the oven to 375°F (190°C).

Place tilapia fillet and asparagus on a baking sheet.

Season with lemon juice, salt, and pepper.

Bake until the tilapia is fully cooked and the asparagus is tender.

## Shrimp and Broccoli Stir-Fry

*Nutritional Information (Approximate):*

Calories: 160

Protein: 25g

Carbohydrates: 6g

Fat: 4g

## Ingredients

4 oz cooked shrimp

1 cup broccoli florets

1/4 cup diced onions

1/4 cup sliced bell peppers (assorted colors)

Low-sodium soy sauce (for flavor)

**Instructions**

In a non-stick skillet, sauté the cooked shrimp, broccoli, onions, and bell peppers until heated through.

Add a dash of low-sodium soy sauce for flavor.

## Turkey and Spinach Stir-Fry

*Nutritional Information (Approximate):*

Calories: 150

Protein: 20g

Carbohydrates: 6g

Fat: 5g

## Ingredients

4 oz lean ground turkey

1 cup fresh spinach

1/4 cup sliced mushrooms

1/4 cup diced tomatoes

Low-sodium soy sauce (for flavor)

## Instructions

In a non-stick skillet, cook the lean ground turkey until fully cooked.

Add fresh spinach, sliced mushrooms, and diced tomatoes to the skillet and sauté until heated through.

Add a dash of low-sodium soy sauce for flavor.

## Baked Cod with Steamed Broccoli

*Nutritional Information (Approximate):*

Calories: 140

Protein: 25g

Carbohydrates: 4g

Fat: 3g

**Ingredients**

4 oz cod fillet

1 cup steamed broccoli florets

Lemon juice (for flavor)

Salt and pepper to taste

**Instructions**

Bake the cod fillet until fully cooked.

Season with lemon juice, salt, and pepper.

Serve with steamed broccoli on the side.

## Beef and Zucchini Noodles

*Nutritional Information (Approximate):*

Calories: 150

Protein: 20g

Carbohydrates: 8g

Fat: 6g

**Ingredients**

4 oz lean beef strips

1 zucchini, spiralized into noodles

1/4 cup diced onions

1/4 cup sliced mushrooms

Low-sodium soy sauce (for flavor)

**Instructions**

In a non-stick skillet, cook the lean beef strips until fully cooked.

In the same skillet, sauté zucchini noodles, diced onions, and sliced mushrooms until heated through.

Add a dash of low-sodium soy sauce for flavor.

## Lemon Herb Grilled Shrimp

*Nutritional Information (Approximate):*

Calories: 140

Protein: 25g

Carbohydrates: 2g

Fat: 4g

## Ingredients

 4 oz grilled shrimp

Fresh herbs (e.g., parsley, dill)

Juice of half a lemon

Salt and pepper to taste

## Instructions

Grill the shrimp until heated through.

Season with fresh herbs, lemon juice, salt, and pepper.

## Chicken and Cabbage Stir-Fry

### Nutritional Information (Approximate):

Calories: 160

Protein: 25g

Carbohydrates: 8g

Fat: 4g

## Ingredients

4 oz cooked chicken breast, sliced

1 cup shredded cabbage

1/4 cup diced onions

1/4 cup sliced bell peppers (assorted colors)

Low-sodium soy sauce (for flavor)

## Instructions

In a non-stick skillet, sauté the cooked chicken breast, shredded cabbage, diced onions, and sliced bell peppers until heated through.

Add a dash of low-sodium soy sauce for flavor.

Tofu and Vegetable Stir-Fry

*Nutritional Information (Approximate):*

Calories: 150

Protein: 15g

Carbohydrates: 10g

Fat: 6g

**Ingredients**

4 oz extra-firm tofu, cubed

1 cup sliced bell peppers (assorted colors)

1 cup sliced zucchini

1/4 cup diced onions

Low-sodium soy sauce (for flavor)

**Instructions**

In a non-stick skillet, cook the tofu until heated through.

Add sliced bell peppers, zucchini, onions, and a dash of low-sodium soy sauce.

Sauté until vegetables are tender.

## Beef and Broccoli with Cauliflower Rice

*Nutritional Information (Approximate):*

Calories: 160

Protein: 20g

Carbohydrates: 8g

Fat: 6g

**Ingredients**

4 oz lean beef strips

1 cup steamed broccoli florets

1 cup cauliflower rice

Low-sodium soy sauce (for flavor)

**Instructions**

In a non-stick skillet, cook the lean beef strips until fully cooked.

Serve with steamed broccoli on one side and cauliflower rice on the other.

Add a dash of low-sodium soy sauce for flavor.

## Grilled Lemon Herb Chicken

*Nutritional Information (Approximate):*

Calories: 150

Protein: 25g

Carbohydrates: 2g

Fat: 4g

**Ingredients**

4 oz grilled chicken breast

Fresh herbs (e.g., basil, thyme)

Juice of half a lemon

Salt and pepper to taste

**Instructions**

Grill the chicken breast until fully cooked.

Season with fresh herbs, lemon juice, salt, and pepper.

## Shrimp and Spinach Salad

*Nutritional Information (Approximate):*

Calories: 140

Protein: 25g

Carbohydrates: 4g

Fat: 3g

**Ingredients**

4 oz cooked shrimp

2 cups fresh spinach

1/4 cup diced tomatoes

1/4 cup sliced cucumbers

Balsamic vinegar (as dressing)

**Instructions**

Place cooked shrimp on a bed of fresh spinach.

Top with diced tomatoes and sliced cucumbers.

Drizzle with balsamic vinegar for dressing.

## Baked Cod with Steamed Green Beans

*Nutritional Information (Approximate):*

Calories: 140

Protein: 25g

Carbohydrates: 4g

Fat: 3g

**Ingredients**

4 oz cod fillet

1 cup steamed green beans

Lemon juice (for flavor)

Salt and pepper to taste

**Instructions**

Bake the cod fillet until fully cooked.

Season with lemon juice, salt, and pepper.

Serve with steamed green beans on the side.

Turkey and Asparagus Stir-Fry

*Nutritional Information (Approximate):*

Calories: 150

Protein: 20g

Carbohydrates: 6g

Fat: 5g

**Ingredients**

4 oz lean ground turkey

1 cup asparagus spears, cut into bite-sized pieces

1/4 cup diced onions

1/4 cup diced bell peppers (assorted colors)

Low-sodium soy sauce (for flavor)

**Instructions**

In a non-stick skillet, cook the lean ground turkey until fully cooked.

Add asparagus, onions, and bell peppers to the skillet and sauté until tender.

Add a dash of low-sodium soy sauce for flavor.

## Lemon Herb Grilled Turkey

*Nutritional Information (Approximate):*

Calories: 150

Protein: 25g

Carbohydrates: 2g

Fat: 4g

**Ingredients**

4 oz grilled turkey breast

Fresh herbs (e.g., rosemary, sage)

Juice of half a lemon

Salt and pepper to taste

**Instructions**

Grill the turkey breast until fully cooked.

Season with fresh herbs, lemon juice, salt, and pepper.

# Chicken and Cabbage Stir-Fry

*Nutritional Information (Approximate):*

Calories: 160

Protein: 25g

Carbohydrates: 8g

Fat: 4g

## Ingredients

4 oz cooked chicken breast, sliced

1 cup shredded cabbage

1/4 cup diced onions

1/4 cup sliced bell peppers (assorted colors)

**Low-sodium soy sauce (for flavor)**

**Instructions**

In a non-stick skillet, sauté the cooked chicken breast, shredded cabbage, diced onions, and sliced bell peppers until heated through.

Add a dash of low-sodium soy sauce for flavor.

## Beef and Cauliflower Rice Stir-Fry

*Nutritional Information (Approximate):*

Calories: 160

Protein: 20g

Carbohydrates: 8g

Fat: 6g

## Ingredients

4 oz lean beef strips

1 cup cauliflower rice

1/4 cup diced onions

1/4 cup sliced mushrooms

Low-sodium soy sauce (for flavor)

## Instructions

In a non-stick skillet, cook the lean beef strips until fully cooked.

Sauté cauliflower rice, diced onions, and sliced mushrooms until heated through.

Add a dash of low-sodium soy sauce for flavor.

## Tofu and Broccoli Stir-Fry

*Nutritional Information (Approximate):*

Calories: 150

Protein: 15g

Carbohydrates: 10g

Fat: 6g

## Ingredients

4 oz extra-firm tofu, cubed

1 cup broccoli florets

1/4 cup diced onions

1/4 cup sliced bell peppers (assorted colors)

Low-sodium soy sauce (for flavor)

**Instructions**

In a non-stick skillet, cook the tofu until heated through.

Add broccoli florets, diced onions, and sliced bell peppers to the skillet and sauté until tender.

Add a dash of low-sodium soy sauce for flavor.

## Grilled Lemon Herb Shrimp

*Nutritional Information (Approximate):*

Calories: 140

Protein: 25g

Carbohydrates: 2g

Fat: 4g

## Ingredients

4 oz grilled shrimp

Fresh herbs (e.g., tarragon, chives)

Juice of half a lemon

Salt and pepper to taste

**Instructions**

Grill the shrimp until heated through.

Season with fresh herbs, lemon juice, salt, and pepper.

## Chicken and Cauliflower Mash

*Nutritional Information (Approximate):*

Calories: 160

Protein: 25g

Carbohydrates: 6g

Fat: 4g

## Ingredients

4 oz grilled chicken breast, sliced

1 cup steamed cauliflower florets

Salt and pepper to taste

Chopped fresh parsley (for garnish)

## Instructions

Grill the chicken breast until fully cooked.

Steam cauliflower florets until tender and mash them.

Serve sliced chicken breast on a bed of cauliflower mash.

Season with salt and pepper, and garnish with chopped fresh parsley.

## DESSERT RECIPES

**Strawberry and Mint Salad**

*Nutritional Information (Approximate):*

Calories: 60

Protein: 1g

Carbohydrates: 14g

Fat: 0g

**Ingredients**

1 cup sliced strawberries

Fresh mint leaves (for garnish)

Stevia or monk fruit sweetener (optional)

**Instructions**

Slice the strawberries and place them in a bowl.

Garnish with fresh mint leaves.

If desired, sweeten with a small amount of stevia or monk fruit sweetener.

# Cinnamon Baked Apple

*Nutritional Information (Approximate):*

Calories: 70

Protein: 0g

Carbohydrates: 18g

Fat: 0g

## Ingredients

1 apple, cored and sliced

1/2 tsp ground cinnamon

Stevia or monk fruit sweetener (optional)

## Instructions

Preheat the oven to 350°F (175°C).

Place apple slices in an oven-safe dish.

Sprinkle with ground cinnamon.

Bake for 15-20 minutes or until the apples are tender.

If desired, sweeten with a small amount of stevia or monk fruit sweetener.

**Mixed Berry Delight**

*Nutritional Information (Approximate):*

Calories: 70

Protein: 2g

Carbohydrates: 15g

Fat: 0g

**Ingredients**

1/2 cup mixed berries (e.g., strawberries, blueberries, raspberries)

A few drops of lemon juice

Stevia or monk fruit sweetener (optional)

**Instructions**

Combine mixed berries in a bowl.

Squeeze a few drops of lemon juice over the berries.

If desired, sweeten with a small amount of stevia or monk fruit sweetener.


## Chilled Lemon Gelato

*Nutritional Information (Approximate):*

Calories: 60

Protein: 2g

Carbohydrates: 10g

Fat: 1g

## Ingredients

1/2 cup Greek yogurt

Zest and juice of half a lemon

Stevia or monk fruit sweetener (optional)

**Instructions**

In a bowl, mix Greek yogurt, lemon zest, and lemon juice.

If desired, sweeten with a small amount of stevia or monk fruit sweetener.

Place the mixture in the freezer until it reaches a gelato-like consistency.

## Cacao-Dusted Strawberries

*Nutritional Information (Approximate):*

Calories: 40

Protein: 1g

Carbohydrates: 10g

Fat: 0g

**Ingredients**

6 strawberries

1 tsp unsweetened cocoa powder

Stevia or monk fruit sweetener (optional)

**Instructions**

Wash and dry the strawberries.

Sprinkle them with unsweetened cocoa powder.

If desired, sweeten with a small amount of stevia or monk fruit sweetener.

## Cinnamon Baked Pear

*Nutritional Information (Approximate):*

Calories: 80

Protein: 1g

Carbohydrates: 20g

Fat: 0g

## Ingredients

1 pear, cored and sliced

1/2 tsp ground cinnamon

Stevia or monk fruit sweetener (optional)

**Instructions**

Preheat the oven to 350°F (175°C).

Place pear slices in an oven-safe dish.

Sprinkle with ground cinnamon.

Bake for 15-20 minutes or until the pears are tender.

If desired, sweeten with a small amount of stevia or monk fruit sweetener.

## Raspberry Sorbet

*Nutritional Information (Approximate):*

Calories: 60

Protein: 1g

Carbohydrates: 15g

Fat: 0g

**Ingredients**

1/2 cup frozen raspberries

A few drops of lemon juice

Stevia or monk fruit sweetener (optional)

**Instructions**

Place frozen raspberries in a blender.

Add a few drops of lemon juice.

If desired, sweeten with a small amount of stevia or monk fruit sweetener.

Blend until smooth and serve as a sorbet.

## Cinnamon and Stevia Baked Grapefruit

*Nutritional Information (Approximate):*

Calories: 50

Protein: 1g

Carbohydrates: 10g

Fat: 0g

**Ingredients**

1/2 grapefruit, halved

1/2 tsp ground cinnamon

Stevia or monk fruit sweetener (optional)

**Instructions**

Preheat the oven to 350°F (175°C).

Sprinkle the grapefruit halves with ground cinnamon.

If desired, sweeten with a small amount of stevia or monk fruit sweetener.

Bake for 15-20 minutes or until the grapefruit is tender.

## Frozen Banana Bites

*Nutritional Information (Approximate):*

Calories: 70

Protein: 2g

Carbohydrates: 18g

Fat: 0g

## Ingredients

1 small banana, sliced into rounds

A few drops of lemon juice

Stevia or monk fruit sweetener (optional)

**Instructions**

In a bowl, toss banana rounds with a few drops of
lemon juice.

If desired, sweeten with a small amount of stevia or
monk fruit sweetener.

Place banana rounds in the freezer until frozen.

## Chocolate-Dipped Strawberries

*Nutritional Information (Approximate):*

Calories: 60

Protein: 1g

Carbohydrates: 15g

Fat: 1g

**Ingredients**

6 strawberries

1 square of unsweetened chocolate

Stevia or monk fruit sweetener (optional)

**Instructions**

Wash and dry the strawberries.

Melt the unsweetened chocolate in a microwave or over a double boiler.

Dip each strawberry into the melted chocolate.

Place them on a tray and let them cool until the chocolate hardens.

If desired, sweeten with a small amount of stevia or monk fruit sweetener.

## Vanilla Almond Pears

*Nutritional Information (Approximate):*

Calories: 80

Protein: 2g

Carbohydrates: 15g

Fat: 2g

## Ingredients

1 pear, cored and sliced

1/4 tsp pure vanilla extract

1 tbsp sliced almonds

Stevia or monk fruit sweetener (optional)

## Instructions

Place pear slices in a bowl.

Drizzle with pure vanilla extract.

If desired, sweeten with a small amount of stevia or monk fruit sweetener.

Top with sliced almonds.

## Berries with Whipped Coconut Cream

*Nutritional Information (Approximate):*

Calories: 90

Protein: 1g

Carbohydrates: 15g

Fat: 4g

**Ingredients**

1/2 cup mixed berries (e.g., raspberries, blackberries)

1/4 cup full-fat coconut milk

Stevia or monk fruit sweetener (optional)

**Instructions**

Chill a can of full-fat coconut milk in the refrigerator for several hours or overnight.

Scoop out the solid coconut cream on top.

Whip the coconut cream with a mixer until light and fluffy.

Serve mixed berries with a dollop of whipped coconut cream.

If desired, sweeten with a small amount of stevia or monk fruit sweetener.

## Lemon Poppy Seed Muffins

*Nutritional Information (Approximate):*

Calories: 80

Protein: 3g

Carbohydrates: 10g

Fat: 3g

**Ingredients**

1 egg white

1 tsp lemon zest

1 tsp lemon juice

1/4 tsp poppy seeds

Stevia or monk fruit sweetener (optional)

**Instructions**

Preheat the oven to 350°F (175°C).

In a bowl, mix the egg white, lemon zest, lemon juice, and poppy seeds.

Pour the mixture into a greased mini muffin tin.

Bake for 10-12 minutes or until a toothpick comes out clean.

If desired, sweeten with a small amount of stevia or monk fruit sweetener.

## Coconut Pineapple Sorbet

*Nutritional Information (Approximate):*

Calories: 70

Protein: 1g

Carbohydrates: 17g

Fat: 1g

## Ingredients

1/2 cup frozen pineapple chunks

2 tbsp unsweetened shredded coconut

Stevia or monk fruit sweetener (optional)

**Instructions**

Place frozen pineapple chunks in a blender.

Add unsweetened shredded coconut.

If desired, sweeten with a small amount of stevia or monk fruit sweetener.

Blend until smooth and serve as a sorbet.

**Chocolate Avocado Pudding**

*Nutritional Information (Approximate):*

Calories: 90

Protein: 2g

Carbohydrates: 9g

Fat: 5g

**Ingredients**

1/2 ripe avocado

1 tbsp unsweetened cocoa powder

Stevia or monk fruit sweetener (optional)

**Instructions**

In a blender, combine the ripe avocado and unsweetened cocoa powder.

If desired, sweeten with a small amount of stevia or monk fruit sweetener.

Blend until smooth.

Chill in the refrigerator before serving.

## Raspberry Lemon Sorbet

*Nutritional Information (Approximate):*

Calories: 70

Protein: 1g

Carbohydrates: 16g

Fat: 0g

**Ingredients**

1/2 cup frozen raspberries

Juice of half a lemon

Stevia or monk fruit sweetener (optional)

**Instructions**

Place frozen raspberries in a blender.

Add the juice of half a lemon.

If desired, sweeten with a small amount of stevia or monk fruit sweetener.

Blend until smooth and serve as a sorbet.

# Cinnamon Baked Banana

## *Nutritional Information (Approximate):*

Calories: 80

Protein: 1g

Carbohydrates: 20g

Fat: 0g

## Ingredients

1 banana

1/2 tsp ground cinnamon

Stevia or monk fruit sweetener (optional)

## Instructions

Preheat the oven to 350°F (175°C).

Place the whole banana in the peel on a baking sheet.

Sprinkle with ground cinnamon.

Bake for 15-20 minutes or until the banana is tender.

If desired, sweeten with a small amount of stevia or monk fruit sweetener.

## Chocolate-Dipped Orange Slices

*Nutritional Information (Approximate):*

Calories: 70

Protein: 1g

Carbohydrates: 15g

Fat: 2g

## Ingredients

4 orange slices

1 square of unsweetened chocolate

Stevia or monk fruit sweetener (optional)

## Instructions

Slice oranges into rounds.

Melt the unsweetened chocolate in a microwave or over a double boiler.

Dip each orange slice into the melted chocolate.

Place them on a tray and let them cool until the chocolate hardens.

If desired, sweeten with a small amount of stevia or monk fruit sweetener.

## Strawberry and Basil Sorbet

*Nutritional Information (Approximate):*

Calories: 70

Protein: 1g

Carbohydrates: 17g

Fat: 0g

**Ingredients**

1/2 cup frozen strawberries

Fresh basil leaves (for flavor)

Stevia or monk fruit sweetener (optional)

**Instructions**

Place frozen strawberries in a blender.

Add fresh basil leaves for a unique flavor twist.

If desired, sweeten with a small amount of stevia or monk fruit sweetener.

Blend until smooth and serve as a sorbet.

# Blueberry Chia Pudding

*Nutritional Information (Approximate):*

Calories: 70

Protein: 2g

Carbohydrates: 15g

Fat: 2g

## Ingredients

1/4 cup chia seeds

1/2 cup unsweetened almond milk

1/2 cup fresh blueberries

Stevia or monk fruit sweetener (optional)

## Instructions

Mix chia seeds and unsweetened almond milk in a bowl.

Let it sit for a few hours to allow chia seeds to absorb the liquid and thicken.

Top with fresh blueberries.

If desired, sweeten with a small amount of stevia or monk fruit sweetener.

# SALAD RECIPES

## Classic Garden Salad

*Nutritional Information (Approximate):*

Calories: 50

Protein: 2g

Carbohydrates: 10g

Fat: 0g

## Ingredients

2 cups mixed salad greens (e.g., lettuce, spinach)

1/4 cup sliced cucumber

1/4 cup sliced tomatoes

1/4 cup sliced bell peppers (assorted colors)

Balsamic vinegar (as dressing)

**Instructions**

Combine salad greens, cucumber, tomatoes, and bell peppers in a bowl.

Drizzle with balsamic vinegar as dressing.

**Spinach and Strawberry Salad**

*Nutritional Information (Approximate):*

Calories: 60

Protein: 2g

Carbohydrates: 12g

Fat: 0g

**Ingredients**

2 cups fresh spinach

1/2 cup sliced strawberries

1/4 cup sliced red onions

Stevia or monk fruit sweetener (optional)

Balsamic vinegar (as dressing)

**Instructions**

Combine fresh spinach, sliced strawberries, and red onions in a bowl.

If desired, sweeten with a small amount of stevia or monk fruit sweetener.

Drizzle with balsamic vinegar as dressing.

## Cucumber and Dill Salad

*Nutritional Information (Approximate):*

Calories: 40

Protein: 1g

Carbohydrates: 8g

Fat: 0g

**Ingredients**

1 cucumber, sliced

1/4 cup diced red onions

Fresh dill (for flavor)

Lemon juice (as dressing)

**Instructions**

Combine sliced cucumber and diced red onions in a bowl.

Season with fresh dill.

Drizzle with lemon juice as dressing.

## Greek Salad

*Nutritional Information (Approximate):*

Calories: 60

Protein: 3g

Carbohydrates: 8g

Fat: 2g

## Ingredients

2 cups mixed salad greens

1/4 cup diced cucumbers

1/4 cup diced tomatoes

1/4 cup diced red onions

1 oz feta cheese (optional)

Kalamata olives (optional)

Balsamic vinegar (as dressing)

**Instructions**

Combine salad greens, cucumbers, tomatoes, red onions, and feta cheese (if desired) in a bowl.

Top with Kalamata olives (if desired).

Drizzle with balsamic vinegar as dressing.

# Grilled Chicken Caesar Salad

## *Nutritional Information (Approximate):*

Calories: 120

Protein: 25g

Carbohydrates: 4g

Fat: 2g

## Ingredients

4 oz grilled chicken breast, sliced

2 cups Romaine lettuce

1 tbsp grated Parmesan cheese

Lemon juice (as dressing)

## Instructions

Place sliced grilled chicken breast on a bed of Romaine lettuce.

Sprinkle with grated Parmesan cheese.

Drizzle with lemon juice as dressing.

## Caprese Salad

*Nutritional Information (Approximate):*

Calories: 80

Protein: 4g

Carbohydrates: 4g

Fat: 6g

## Ingredients

1 cup cherry tomatoes

1 oz fresh mozzarella cheese, sliced

Fresh basil leaves (for flavor)

Balsamic vinegar (as dressing)

## Instructions

Combine cherry tomatoes and fresh mozzarella cheese slices in a bowl.

Season with fresh basil leaves.

Drizzle with balsamic vinegar as dressing.

## Tuna Salad

*Nutritional Information (Approximate):*

Calories: 100

Protein: 20g

Carbohydrates: 4g

Fat: 2g

## Ingredients

4 oz canned tuna, drained

1/4 cup diced cucumbers

1/4 cup diced tomatoes

1/4 cup diced red onions

Lemon juice (as dressing)

**Instructions**

Combine canned tuna, diced cucumbers, tomatoes, and red onions in a bowl.

Drizzle with lemon juice as dressing.

**Waldorf Salad**

*Nutritional Information (Approximate):*

Calories: 80

Protein: 1g

Carbohydrates: 12g

Fat: 3g

**Ingredients**

1/2 apple, diced

1/4 cup chopped celery

1/4 cup chopped walnuts

A few drops of lemon juice

Stevia or monk fruit sweetener (optional)

**Instructions**

Combine diced apple, chopped celery, and chopped walnuts in a bowl.

Squeeze a few drops of lemon juice over the mixture.

If desired, sweeten with a small amount of stevia or monk fruit sweetener.

## Avocado and Tomato Salad

***Nutritional Information (Approximate):***

Calories: 70

Protein: 2g

Carbohydrates: 4g

Fat: 5g

## Ingredients

1 avocado, diced

1/2 cup diced tomatoes

1/4 cup diced red onions

Fresh cilantro (for flavor)

Lemon juice (as dressing)

## Instructions

Combine diced avocado, diced tomatoes, and diced red onions in a bowl.

Season with fresh cilantro.

Drizzle with lemon juice as dressing.

## Broccoli and Almond Salad

*Nutritional Information (Approximate):*

Calories: 70

Protein: 3g

Carbohydrates: 8g

Fat: 3g

## Ingredients

1 cup steamed broccoli florets

1 tbsp sliced almonds

1/4 cup diced red onions

A few drops of lemon juice

Stevia or monk fruit sweetener (optional)

**Instructions**

Combine steamed broccoli florets, sliced almonds, and diced red onions in a bowl.

Squeeze a few drops of lemon juice over the mixture.

If desired, sweeten with a small amount of stevia or monk fruit sweetener.

## Tofu and Spinach Salad

*Nutritional Information (Approximate):*

Calories: 70

Protein: 10g

Carbohydrates: 6g

Fat: 3g

**Ingredients**

4 oz extra-firm tofu, cubed

2 cups fresh spinach

1/4 cup sliced cucumbers

1/4 cup sliced cherry tomatoes

Balsamic vinegar (as dressing)

**Instructions**

In a non-stick skillet, sauté the cubed tofu until heated through.

Combine fresh spinach, sliced cucumbers, and cherry tomatoes in a bowl.

Add the sautéed tofu on top.

Drizzle with balsamic vinegar as dressing.

## Beef and Bean Salad

*Nutritional Information (Approximate):*

Calories: 120

Protein: 15g

Carbohydrates: 10g

Fat: 2g

**Ingredients**

4 oz lean ground beef

1 cup green beans, steamed and cut into bite-sized pieces

1/4 cup diced red onions

1/4 cup sliced bell peppers (assorted colors)

Lemon juice (as dressing)

**Instructions**

In a non-stick skillet, cook the lean ground beef until fully cooked.

Combine steamed green beans, diced red onions, and sliced bell peppers in a bowl.

Add the cooked ground beef on top.

Drizzle with lemon juice as dressing.

## Salmon and Asparagus Salad

*Nutritional Information (Approximate):*

Calories: 140

Protein: 20g

Carbohydrates: 4g

Fat: 5g

## Ingredients

4 oz grilled salmon fillet, flaked

1 cup steamed asparagus

1/4 cup sliced cherry tomatoes

Fresh dill (for flavor)

Balsamic vinegar (as dressing)

## Instructions

Grill the salmon fillet until fully cooked, then flake it.

Combine steamed asparagus, sliced cherry tomatoes, and flaked salmon in a bowl.

Season with fresh dill.

Drizzle with balsamic vinegar as dressing.

## Shrimp and Avocado Salad

*Nutritional Information (Approximate):*

Calories: 90

Protein: 12g

Carbohydrates: 4g

Fat: 4g

**Ingredients**

4 oz cooked shrimp

1/2 avocado, diced

2 cups mixed salad greens

Fresh cilantro (for flavor)

Lemon juice (as dressing)

**Instructions**

Place cooked shrimp on a bed of mixed salad greens.

Top with diced avocado.

Season with fresh cilantro.

Drizzle with lemon juice as dressing.

# Chicken and Zucchini Salad

## *Nutritional Information (Approximate):*

Calories: 90

Protein: 15g

Carbohydrates: 6g

Fat: 2g

## Ingredients

4 oz grilled chicken breast, sliced

1 cup sliced zucchini

1/4 cup diced red onions

Fresh thyme (for flavor)

Balsamic vinegar (as dressing)

**Instructions**

Grill the chicken breast until fully cooked, then slice it.

Combine sliced zucchini, diced red onions, and sliced chicken in a bowl.

Season with fresh thyme.

Drizzle with balsamic vinegar as dressing.

## Tofu and Cabbage Salad

*Nutritional Information (Approximate):*

Calories: 70

Protein: 9g

Carbohydrates: 6g

Fat: 2g

## Ingredients

4 oz extra-firm tofu, cubed

1 cup shredded cabbage

1/4 cup diced red onions

Fresh mint leaves (for flavor)

Lemon juice (as dressing)

## Instructions

In a non-stick skillet, sauté the cubed tofu until heated through.

Combine shredded cabbage, diced red onions, and sautéed tofu in a bowl.

Season with fresh mint leaves.

Drizzle with lemon juice as dressing.

## Turkey and Mushroom Salad

*Nutritional Information (Approximate):*

Calories: 110

Protein: 15g

Carbohydrates: 6g

Fat: 3g

## Ingredients

4 oz lean ground turkey

1 cup sliced mushrooms

1/4 cup diced red onions

Fresh rosemary (for flavor)

Balsamic vinegar (as dressing)

## Instructions

In a non-stick skillet, cook the lean ground turkey until fully cooked.

Add sliced mushrooms and diced red onions to the skillet and sauté until tender.

Season with fresh rosemary.

Drizzle with balsamic vinegar as dressing.

## Tuna and Radish Salad

*Nutritional Information (Approximate):*

Calories: 90

Protein: 15g

Carbohydrates: 4g

Fat: 2g

**Ingredients**

4 oz canned tuna, drained

1/4 cup sliced radishes

2 cups mixed salad greens

Fresh parsley (for flavor)

Lemon juice (as dressing)

**Instructions**

Combine canned tuna, sliced radishes, and mixed salad greens in a bowl.

Season with fresh parsley.

Drizzle with lemon juice as dressing.

# Beef and Spinach Salad

*Nutritional Information (Approximate):*

Calories: 120

Protein: 15g

Carbohydrates: 6g

Fat: 4g

## Ingredients

4 oz lean ground beef

2 cups fresh spinach

1/4 cup sliced mushrooms

1/4 cup diced red onions

Fresh oregano (for flavor)

Balsamic vinegar (as dressing)

**Instructions**

In a non-stick skillet, cook the lean ground beef until fully cooked.

Combine fresh spinach, sliced mushrooms, diced red onions, and cooked ground beef in a bowl.

Season with fresh oregano.

Drizzle with balsamic vinegar as dressing.

## Chicken and Broccoli Salad

*Nutritional Information (Approximate):*

Calories: 100

Protein: 15g

Carbohydrates: 6g

Fat: 3g

**Ingredients**

4 oz grilled chicken breast, sliced

1 cup steamed broccoli florets

1/4 cup sliced cherry tomatoes

Fresh basil leaves (for flavor)

Lemon juice (as dressing)

**Instructions**

Grill the chicken breast until fully cooked, then slice it.

Combine steamed broccoli florets, sliced cherry tomatoes, sliced chicken, and fresh basil leaves in a bowl.

Drizzle with lemon juice as dressing.

# Chapter 5: Staying Safe on the HCG Diet

There are a number of potential health problems and dangers connected to the HCG (Human Chorionic Gonadotropin) diet. The very low-calorie diet it necessitates is a significant hindrance. During the low-calorie period, you may only be allowed 500 to 800 calories per day. Extreme calorie restriction has been linked to tiredness, malnutrition, and other health issues.

Although it is claimed that this diet will prevent muscle loss while relying on fat stores for fuel, extreme calorie restriction can have this effect. Furthermore, there is scant evidence that the diet is effective, and this is not universally acknowledged by medical specialists.

The HCG diet emphasizes speedy weight loss at the expense of health, which may lead to gallstones and other problems. Sagging skin is another possible side effect of rapid weight loss.

People on the HCG diet may be at risk for nutritional deficiencies due to the restricted dietary options and low calorie intake. Hormone replacement therapy (HRT) using HCG injections or dietary drops may alter hormone levels, which might influence menstrual cycles in women and hormonal balance in males.

This low-calorie diet may be difficult to maintain due to the possibility of feeling hungry all the time. This, in turn, may lead to binge eating after stopping the diet. A lack of essential nutrients may be to blame for the hair loss experienced by certain people.

As the HCG diet does not encourage permanent lifestyle changes, it is typical for lost weight to be regained after completion. In addition, there is no guarantee that HCG products are safe or controlled, therefore it is important to verify their authenticity and only use them under the care of a doctor.

The HCG diet is a highly contentious and restricted weight loss method with possible hazards connected to extreme calorie restriction, fast weight loss, and hormonal impacts. For healthy, long-term weight loss and improved well-being, it's best to discuss options with a medical expert.

## Getting Medical Supervision

In the context of the HCG diet, monitoring and medical supervision play an essential role. Before starting this diet, it's vital to contact with a healthcare expert who can assess your health, identify any dangers, and discuss any underlying medical issues or drugs you may be taking. This evaluation will help us figure out if the HCG diet is a good fit for you.

The implications of excessive calorie restriction on your health and any potential adverse effects may be discussed with your doctor. If you have a medical condition that necessitates changes to the diet for your safety, they can tailor the diet plan to match your individual health demands.

Regular medical check-ins during the diet enable for the tracking of your progress and the early diagnosis of undesirable effects or issues. This allows for fast action in the event that the diet has to be modified or stopped altogether.

In order to prevent nutritional deficiencies, it is crucial to have medical monitoring to ensure that the diet includes vital nutrients, vitamins, and minerals despite the low calorie consumption. Healthcare providers can monitor your drug regimen and make modifications to your dose if required when drug interactions are discovered.

Doctors may keep an eye on HCG dieters' hormone levels and treat any imbalances or unwanted effects that crop up while on the diet. Healthcare experts can advise patients on how to deal with symptoms including tiredness, hair loss, and mood swings.

When combined with a nutritious diet and regular exercise, medical supervision can help dieters successfully return to a healthy weight and lifestyle. Health care providers may educate their patients about the risks of fad diets like the HCG diet and the benefits of more moderate, long-term approaches to weight management. To sum up, your health and safety should come first, so talk to your doctor before beginning the HCG diet or any other drastic weight reduction program.

## Setbacks and How to Solve Them

### Extreme calorie restriction

Extreme calorie restriction, as in the HCG diet, can cause hunger, fatigue, and mood swings. Water and herbal teas are great options for this since they help keep you hydrated and hence less hungry. You can further reduce your daily calorie consumption by eating smaller, more often meals consisting of the permitted items.

## Not Enough Food Options

Because of the diet's limitations, mealtimes may become routine and boring. To overcome this obstacle, try various combinations of spices and flavors. Get creative with the authorized items, such as finding novel ways to prepare and combine them to make your meals interesting.

## Constraints Imposed By Culture and Habitual Behavior

Social gatherings and activities may provide obstacles, since you may need to avoid certain meals and beverages. To get over this difficulty, prepare ahead of time for social events by sticking to the diet or selecting healthy choices that are in line with the HCG diet guidelines. Sharing your food limits with loved ones will help you get their understanding and support.

## Potential Side Effects

While on the HCG diet, some people may feel tired, lose their hair, or suffer shifts in their mood. Seek advice from a medical expert on how to deal with these unwanted consequences. They may advise you on how to deal with certain concerns and keep an eye on your general health while you eat.

## Making the Right Lifestyle Choices

Adopting a healthy lifestyle is crucial for your entire well-being and long-term health. It's a set of decisions that can improve your physical and emotional health while also aiding in weight maintenance. Maintaining a healthy diet should be your first priority. Eat a wide range of fresh produce, whole grains, lean proteins, and healthy fats, while cutting back on processed foods, sugary snacks, and salt.

Regular physical exercise is another cornerstone of a healthy lifestyle. To increase cardiovascular health, muscle strength, and flexibility, it's important to do both aerobic workouts like walking or running and strength training. It's crucial to take in sufficient fluids via water consumption throughout the day. Keep yourself well-hydrated by limiting your intake of sugary drinks and coffee.

Get plenty of shut-eye; it'll do wonders for your body and mind. Get between seven and nine hours of sleep nightly. Managing stress is also important. Mindfulness, meditation, deep breathing exercises, and relaxing hobbies are all great ways to reduce stress.

Moderation in alcohol use is encouraged since heavy drinking has been linked to several health problems. Furthermore, as smoking is a main source of avoidable illnesses and health issues, adopt a tobacco-free lifestyle by not smoking and reducing exposure to secondhand smoke.

The best way to keep tabs on your health, stave off possible problems, and get preventative treatment is to schedule regular checks with your doctor. Finally, when you feel you need it, reach out for help with your mental health. Seeking help from a therapist, counselor, or other mental health professional is one option. Maintain healthy friendships and relationships since they have a profound effect on your psychological and emotional well-being. By integrating these healthy lifestyle choices, you may boost your quality of life and overall health.

# Chapter 6: Final Notes

Keep in mind that making healthy choices is an ongoing process. How you eat, deal with stress, and stay active are just a few of the everyday decisions that may have a major effect on your health and happiness.

It is essential to put your health first by adhering to a regimen of healthy eating, regular exercise, sufficient rest, and stress management. A healthy lifestyle also includes limiting one's intake of alcoholic beverages and refraining from using tobacco products.

Preventative and screening measures used as part of regular checkups allow for the early detection and treatment of health problems. It's equally crucial to attention to your mental health, seeking assistance and therapy when required, and maintaining strong connections for emotional well-being.

The road to health is rarely a straight line, and it's OK to seek advice from medical doctors, nutritionists, and psychologists so that you may find the best plan of action for you. Keep in mind that slow, steady shifts are usually more effective and enduring in the long run than drastic, hasty ones.

An investment in your future health and happiness is what adopting a healthy lifestyle is all about. You may proactively work toward a longer, healthier, and more satisfying life by including these options into your routine.